SIXTY STEPS TO REDUCE TENSION

CRESTLINE BOOKS

This book is dedicated to all those who see values in the uses of alternative theraphy in solving daily health and social problems

Contents

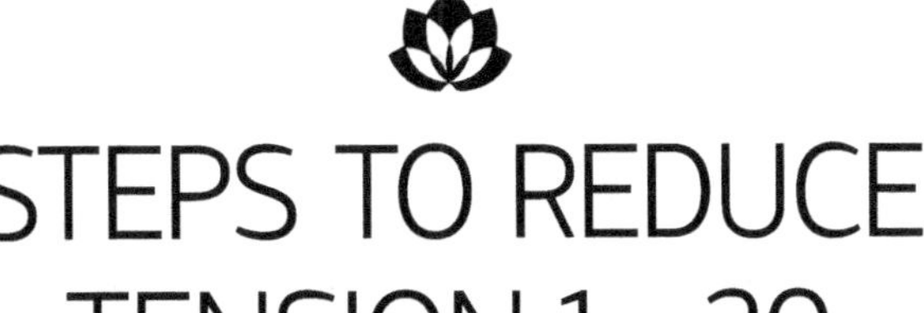

CHAPTER ONE

STEPS TO REDUCE TENSION 1 - 20

1, Identify the real cause of stress.

2, Events causing stress should be noted down and analyzed once a month.

3, Your reactions to each stressful event should be recollected and compared with one another.

4, Should not give immediate responses to the stressful event, always take little time to think.

5, If any tension comes ask your inner man(Mind)for a solution, he is more intelligent than you.

6, Past is past always concentrate on future events and gather courage and willpower.

7, Need not bother about your loss, but find out the reason for it and try to solve it.

8, Face all situations with confidence.

9, Keep faith in God and worship him.

10, Always hope for the best.

11, Always keep a positive approach.

12, Before doing anything plan a solution to face a negative situation.

13, Should not live only for money.

14, Help the poor people.

15, Visit the sick people and give them moral support.

16, Whenever you are tensed take a deep breath and relax.

17, If you are tensed countdown from 100 to 1.

18, If any stress comes look at the beautiful picture kept on the wall.

19, Keep some flowers in the room and have a look.

20, Practise breathing exercises regularly.

CHAPTER TWO

STEPS TO REDUCE TENSION 21-40

21, Keep little time for yoga and meditation.

22, Aromatherapy is good to relax the mind.

23, If you are tense make a surprise call to your old friend.

24, When you are tense think about others who suffer from more serious problems.

25, Keep close contact with your family and share the problems with them.

26, Go for pleasure trips with the family members.

27, Avoid sedentary life, always mingle with others.

28Always approach others with a smile.

29, Laughing and sharing jokes with others will make you relaxed.

30, When you are tense visit your close friend or relative.

31, If any stressful event comes discuss it with your intimate friend.

32, Spend little time with your kids and join their plays.

33, If you get time go for a healthy discussion on any interesting topic.

34, Always politely approach people.

35, Maximum attempts should be made to reduce enemies.

36, Keep a routine for your activities.

37, Never postpone the work.

38, Sound sleep is very essential to relax your mind and body.

39, Always prefer a room with fresh air.

40, Get up early in the morning.

CHAPTER THREE

STEPS TO REDUCE TENSION 41-60

40. Avoid cabbage odor by adding vinegar to the cooking water. 41. Skunk odor: remove from pets by rubbing fur with vinegar.

42. Paint adheres better to galvanized metal that has been wiped with vinegar.

43. Pets' drinking water: add vinegar to eliminate odor and encourage shiny fur.

44. For the fluffy meringue: beat 3 egg whites with a teaspoon of vinegar.

45. Pie crust: add 1 tablespoon vinegar to your pastry recipe for an exceptional crust.

46. Half a teaspoon per quart of patching plaster allows you more time to work the plaster before it hardens.

47. Prevent discoloration of peeled potatoes by adding a few drops of vinegar to the water. They will keep fresh for days in the fridge.

48. Poultry water: add vinegar to increase egg production and to produce tender meat.

49. Preserve peppers: put freshly picked peppers in a sterilized jar and finish filling with boiling vinegar.

50. Olives and pimentos will keep indefinitely if covered with vinegar and refrigerated.

51. Add 1 tsp. vinegar to the cooking water for fluffier rice. 52. Add vinegar to laundry rinse water: removes all soap and prevents yellowing.

53. After shampoo hair rinse: 1-ounce apple cider vinegar in 1 quart of distilled water.

54. For a shiny crust on homemade bread and rolls: just before they have finished baking, take them out, brush crusts with vinegar, return to the oven to finish baking.

55. Homemade sour cream: blend together 1 cup cottage cheese, 1/4 cup skim milk and 1 tsp. vinegar.

56. Boil vinegar and water in pots to remove stains. 57. Remove berry stains from hands with vinegar.

57. Remove berry stains from hands with vinegar.

58. Prevent sugaring by mixing a drop of vinegar in the cake icing. 59. Cold vinegar relieves sunburn.

60. When boiling meat, add a spoonful of vinegar to the water to make it more tender.

61. Marinate tough meat in vinegar overnight to tenderize. 62. A strength tonic: combine raw eggs, vinegar, and black pepper. Blend well.

63. Douche: 2 to 4 ounces of vinegar in 2 quarts of warm water.

CHAPTER FOUR

Bad Habits You Need to Stop to Improve Your Work Life

You're on a self-improvement mission – good for you! But, before you make a big list of things you can do to improve your life, you should start by looking at the bad habits you need to stop. We all have bad habits and they can all interfere with us being the best we can be. We often feel comfortable doing the same things day after day, but you might not realize that some of these habits can interfere with you being productive and they can even harm your work life.

#1 Stop smoking

If you could inhale productivity like you inhale cigarette smoke, but we can't. What happens is your concentration will decrease after you have a cigarette and so will your productivity. Worse, if you are anxious for your next cigarette your concentration also falters. If you want to be more productive and live a healthier life, you need to quit smoking.

#2 Make the Right Music Choices

The music you would listen to during a workout is going to be much different than the music you listen to while you work. Choose music you like and enjoy and your brain will increase the production of dopamine, which will make you excited rather than focused. So while you are at work, choose ambient music. Avoid music that you are familiar with where you will get distracted singing the words.

#3 No More Than 4 Cups of Coffee

Most of us love our coffee. When you know the right amounts of coffee to drink your brain will be stimulated by it – the areas of concentration, attention, and planning can benefit with approximately 400 mg or 4 cups of coffee a day. However, if you drink more than that it can have the opposite effect and cause you to be irritable, restless, and anxious.

#4 Divide Learning and Working

If you want to develop and increase your skills, learning is vital. Learn what you can and put that to practice. However, you can't let learning interfere with working, as this will hurt your self-improvement. Instead, set aside times or days where learning will be your focus, and then it will not interfere with your work.

#5 Limit Your Rewards

You finish a task. You feel it was difficult and so you deserve a break – that's the reward you give yourself. While it might certainly be the case if you take one reward in the morning and one in the afternoon. That's it, no matter how efficient you are for the day.

When you recognize your bad habits and turn them into good habits, you are well on your way to being more productive.

CHAPTER FIVE

How You Can Achieve Your Inner Peace

If inner peace seems elusive and unattainable, far away or unreal you aren't alone. Most of us feel that way at one time or another. Part of your self-improvement plan can be to learn how to achieve inner peace. It will be a skill that will help you throughout life. You will be calm during times of stress and during situations that need your immediate attention. One thing you need to always remember – to achieve inner peace is to recognize it is defined by outer circumstances. Let's look at the steps you can take.

#1 Simplify

Keeping your life simple will contribute to your inner peace because it directs your energy to a single point. Toss out everything that holds you back. That includes friends and acquaintances who drain you and in return give you nothing. Remember quality over quantity. Keep it simple stay focused.

#2 Be in the Present

The only time that matters is the present because it's the only time that exists. That past was, the present is now and the future will be the present. You have no control over the future, nor can you predict it. So focus on what you do have control over - the present. Give it your best and live

#3 Express Your Gratitude

Take a minute to recognize just how fortunate you are. Your mind may tend to wonder and desire something different. But consider this – more than 80 percent of the world lives on less than $10 a day. Where do you fit into this? Chances are in comparison you are living like a King. Your mind is your worst enemy. Remember, should you get what you desire, you'll only be desiring something else soon. So be grateful for what you have.

#4 Try on Someone Else's Point of View

Your point of view isn't the only one. Don't treat it like it's the law. Be ready to let it go. Don't go to battle over your point of view for the reality is that it is no more than your opinion. If you find yourself in the wrong, be gracious and acknowledge that.

#5 This too Shall Pass

Everything that comes will pass. Time is generous and indifferent. What is dark today may be glorious tomorrow. Everything perishes – everyone perishes. Nothing is forever. Time will heal the deepest wounds. Since whatever is going on today will pass, sometimes the best solution is simply to let it go. Tomorrow is another day – a fresh start.

#6 Smile

Smile – it can do wonders for your spirit and the spirit of others. It can soften hearts and change moods. Smiling is connected to love. You can't smile and be angry or jealous at the same time. Smiling makes you feel calm, happy, and loved.

CHAPTER SIX

We all go through highs and lows in our life. Sometimes it takes the lows for us to decide it's time to focus on some self-improvement. You might be feeling rejected, down, sad, even a little depressed. Remember this – when life is in turmoil, what you need to do is 'smile' and not get caught up in all the negativity. You can use these tough times as a time to learn. Turmoil just isn't a reason for you to stop living.

It's inevitable. You are going to face heartaches and problems throughout your life. These too shall pass. There are some things you can do so that you can come out the other side unscathed. You might be going through tough times right now, but it isn't going to last forever. Things will change, they will get better – keep telling yourself this. No matter what the problem, what turmoil you are facing, this too shall pass. At some point, you will look back and recognize the lesson that you were meant to learn.

In a few years, what's going on will be nothing but a memory. It won't matter. You might even look back and laugh or you might be incredibly thankful for what looked like a terrible ordeal at the time because what came out of it was good and it made you stronger. No matter what is going on in your life, keep in mind that much of what is going on right now will make up just a small percentage of your life. So, instead of letting it pull you into the darkness, think of what you can do to stay focused and strong. What can you do today, in your life that will make positive changes?

Life has plenty of beautiful moments but there is also pain as we grow and it is that pain that will make you stronger. You will endure the pain because you understand that at the end of the day it will be worth it. You will learn how to overcome the pain – that will be part of your self-improvement plan. From the pain, you will morph into a beautiful human being.

What you do need to remember is that the negativity of others isn't your problem. You can be sure that over time there are going to be many people who let you down. During your difficult times, you will know who your real friends are. What you won't need is the negativity of others who leave you feeling worse than you already do. You want to have friends who lift you, lift your spirits, even when your world seems to be collapsing.

Finally, remember, life is full of highs and lows. You can't have one without the other. Your world is ever-changing and your self-improvement can happen during both highs and lows.